MY TURNING POINT

BEFORE MIGRATING TO THE UK (A TRUE LIFE EXPERIENCE OF A BLACK NURSE)

CHINAZO ELIZABETH EGWUH

Copyright © 2022 CHINAZO ELIZABETH EGWUH

All rights reserved.
No part of this book may be reproduced, or stored in a retrieval system, or transmitted in any form or by any means, electronic, mechanical, photocopying, recording, or otherwise, without express written permission of the publisher.

ISBN-9798409467487

CONTENTS

Dedication

Acknowledgments

Introduction

Chapter One: The Beginning of the End

Chapter Two: Getting it Right

Chapter Three: Challenges of Relocation

Chapter Four: The Silver Lining

Chapter Five: The Nesting Phase

Chapter Six: Turning Point

Chapter Seven: Family Reunion

Conclusion

DEDICATION

This book is dedicated to Almighty God and to my dear readers aspiring for greater heights.

ACKNOWLEDGMENTS

I sincerely appreciate all who supported me in every way, as I went through this process. This page will not contain your names if I begin to write all of them down one by one. Thank you all for your support and prayers as I continue to fulfill purpose. God bless you.

I specially want to appreciate my husband, Onyebuchi Egwuh for his encouragement even when I almost gave up.

CONTENTS

Dedication

Acknowledgments

Introduction

Chapter One: The Beginning of the End

Chapter Two: Getting it Right

Chapter Three: Challenges of Relocation

Chapter Four: The Silver Lining

Chapter Five: The Nesting Phase

Chapter Six: Turning Point

Chapter Seven: Family Reunion

Conclusion

INTRODUCTION

"What you put into life is what you get out of it."
Clint Eastwood

You may have come across the above quote before now. Maybe you once heard it from your colleague at work while dishing out advice on how you could finish up a task and on time. You might have flipped through it while skimming through that motivational book your neighbor gave to you as a birthday gift, and perhaps you have never given much thought to it.

Personally, I am at a point in my life where I can boldly say that life has given me everything I put into it; I'm living my dream life! I'm at my sixty moments! However, it wouldn't be completely honest if I declared that life is full of roses. I never had to pick roses from the garden of life. Every part of my life's story comes with a fair share of roses and thorns. Interestingly, this is not to make you roll your eyes at another boring, usual "Grass to Grace" story neatly tucked between books on every bookshelf. What I am about sharing with you in this book is my life, my journey, and the story of my becoming.

Success is a journey. Every individual has his or her definition of success as well as the road map to attaining their destination. For some, success could be finishing grade school, owning houses and properties, buying exotic cars, securing a lucrative job, having enough money in your bank account. It could mean a different thing for different folks. What matters are the processes involved in your pursuit of success. What is your approach to success? How do you define success? Will your end justify the means? I consciously carved out a path for myself early in life.

There were moments where it seemed as if I had lost my way, but I found my way back eventually. It's like going through a journey and mistakenly loses your road map, but fortunately the signs and traces on the way helped you to get you safely to your desired destination.

Relocating to the UK is one of the phases of my life that will remain significant in my journey of success. The joys, downfalls, hard work, sleepless nights, money spent and my resilience all summed up my struggles as a young woman striving to make her life better.

In this book, I will share everything about my life, from my childhood to coming to the UK as a black woman and a foreign nurse. I will hold your hands and walk you through the processes of my journey towards the relocation and settling in the UK, as I leave you to pick up the information and encouragement that you need. I wish that you have the most refreshing experience as you come with me on this journey.Let's go!

CHAPTER ONE

THE BEGINNING OF THE END

"The first step towards getting somewhere is to decide you are not going to stay where you are" – John Pierpont Morgan.

A new beginning means a fresh start and all the amazing possibilities it could bring along with it. Every human being on earth has his unique beginnings that tell their stories: we all started from somewhere. Being born is a beginning and your possibilities start to count from that moment. One wonderful thing about beginnings is that it has an end; it does not allow you to remain where you are, thereby creating ample room for growth and expansion.

There was a cemented board at the back of my mother's drugstore. It was a huge part of my memories growing up in Nigeria, and as expected it formed a solid plank of my beginning. I was born into a middle-class family. I was born between two sisters. Growing up, my parents tried all they could to make sure all our needs were met. I grew up in a family filled with laughter and contentment, as we did a lot of things together. My Dad was our home teacher.

Every education I got now started from the cemented board behind my Mum's drugstore. We would come back from school every afternoon, and would sight my Dad waiting with chalk and piles of Newspapers, otherwise known as dailies, ready for us after lunch. I started mastering words and calculations at a very tender age and grew up setting higher bars or standards for myself.

When it comes to career, I never dreamt of becoming a nurse as a child. And when I decided to become a Nurse, I knew immediately that I wanted something better, and everything I did from that moment was by my goal.

Family is important in the life of every (growing) child. The kind of family a child grows up in determines his or her development. I grew up having lots of extended family members coming to live with us. Most of them were supportive, while some were not. My parents entrusted us in their care, but some of them deliberately molested me. Thankfully, it was the work of providence that I narrowly escaped their snare. I understand that a lot of parents trust their family members to care for their kids, especially when they are your family members. But then, the world is becoming a strange place. It is no longer what it used to be. Therefore, parents must exercise caution as regards in whose hands they entrust the care of their children. Be sure of the people you are entrusting the care of your kids, and do not hesitate to take legal actions when some people have crossed some boundaries regarding your children or wards.

In as much as it's not the fault of the child or the parents when a child is molested, there are precautions you must take as parents towards your child, such as teaching them how and when to speak up; teach them about their private parts and their functions; tell them their body belongs to them and no one else; never shush them when they try to speak up. Last but not least, always be ready to detect their reactions or mood swings, especially when they are around a particular family member. A good percentage of children have been affected by abuse which has the ability to disrupt the actualization of their dreams. In all, children should be protected at all costs and given the freedom to grow and become who they want to be in life.

Once I decided I would become a Nurse, all I did was find ways to achieve my dreams and become the best version of myself. Being a Nurse in Nigeria can be quite overwhelming. I have experienced firsthand the situations and challenges of Nurses in Nigeria, such as:

- Lack of mentorship and work motivation.
- Low pay rates, as compared to their counterparts.
- Presence of Auxiliary Nurses that deface the noble profession of Nursing.

The above challenges could drive a well-trained nurse crazy and make her forget the core ethics of nursing, which is the utmost care of patients. Those challenges affected me, but I reacted to them differently. My experiences rather pushed me to think out of the box in search of better opportunities. I wanted a place where I would be respected and paid well for my services. I started doing lots of research and seeking information on how to relocate to developed countries and practice there as a Nurse. I applied for AVANT but did not meet their requirements. I didn't know then about the UK relocation process until I read a letter written to young and newly qualified nurses in the Nigeria by one great nurse in the UK, Emeka by name. It provoked in me the need to aspire higher and seek greener pastures as a nurse in the UK. At first, I was not interested, as I was already discouraged by the initial disappointment, but I decided to try again.

You will never know the outcome of anything until you try. I gathered reliable information and got sources and links that would help me get a nursing job in the UK. Note that if you ever find yourself as a young individual trying to get jobs in the UK, you must work twice as hard and also be patient. There are lots of things you have to do while aiming for a job in the UK. They include: writing series of exams; registering for and applying to lots of associations and boards; sourcing for vacancies, and most importantly finding a reliable and trustworthy agencies. There are lots of scammers out there that are ready to mislead and run you dry. Please be sure to do your research before giving anyone your hard-earned money.

In the next chapter, I will be giving detailed procedures and information as regards relocating to the UK and all you need to know and do while sourcing for reliable information to realise your goal.

See you there!!!

CHAPTER TWO

GETTING IT RIGHT

"It is not about being right, it's about getting it right" – Elizabeth Spelke

Trying out something entirely different in your life does not come easy. There got to be lots of changes and sacrifices you need to make to achieve a certain feat. However, with determination and hard work in the bag you can always achieve your goals, however impossible it may look.

International English Language Test (IELTS) as a key Requirement for People Aspiring to Relocate to the UK

My relocation preparation was an eye-opener and an introduction to a new phase of my life. The first and important thing you must do while trying to get a nursing job in the UK is writing and acing IELTS. (IELTS translates as International English Language Test), a compulsory English test that is required for most relocation. It may sound so simple at first because it's just English. People would say, just English? The results humble some people.

You may have thought that English Language test at Secondary School level won't be a big deal. Nah!! It's not as easy as you think *mi amor*. Now you know what IELTS is, if you are looking forward to writing it, you must learn to study from the beginning to the end. Most times, it requires going for extra classes. Know that, if you are relocating as a nurse to the UK, writing and passing the IELTS exam will qualify you for the Nursing and Midwifery Council (NMC) the UK. This in the bag, you can proceed to other stages of the relocation processes.

My Personal Experience with International English Language Test (IELTS)

After registering for the IELTS exam in 2018, I started intense preparations immediately. Due to lack of funds, I couldn't register for extra classes. The implication was that I had to teach myself and work as twice as hard. I engaged the use of YouTube videos from recommendable tutors with positive reviews. YouTube tutors like Jay and IELTS UP are highly recommendable if you are looking forward to writing IELTS. I also did a review with Simon IELTS, who scored and gave me corrections. I studied past questions and past videos of past IELTS students as well.

Preparing for the IELTS exam without the help of a private tutor requires lots of energy and attention, especially when you are new to the system. I was scared because I had registered for this exam with good money and wouldn't want it to go down the drain. You register and sit for IELTS only, once, and if you fail a sitting you will have to register again with MONEY. In 2019 when I enrolled for IELTS examination, it was about #70,000 to #80,000. Imagine not passing the exam after at least two sittings. You know how much must have gone down the drain.

I sat for my first IELTS exams on 6 May, 2019. Everything was going well and flowing smoothly as expected on the exam day.

I prepared well for the exam. *Yoooo!!! I didn't come to joke!* Surprisingly, however, I failed the exam. Yes, I failed my first IELTS exams and I couldn't breathe for few seconds, because I was so sure the outcome would gladden my heart.

Now, let me explain something briefly: The IELTS exam is divided into two modules which are academic and general. The only difference between these two modules is that the reading and writing sections are slightly different. The IELTS exam is further divided into four sections:

1. The Writing Section
2. The Reading Section
3. The Speaking Section
4. The Listening Section

The Writing Section

The writing section involves narrating or describing certain essays that would be given to you. This section lasts for 60 minutes.

The Speaking Section

This section involves an interview with a trained IELTS examiner, and it lasts for 11 to 14 minutes.

The Reading Section

This section involves solving questions from three different comprehension texts. This section lasts for 60 minutes.

The Listening Section

This section involves listening to different voice notes and answering questions based on the voice notes. This is the trickiest and most crucial part of the IELTS exam. If you don't give this section your absolute attention and best, you may not scale through it. The listening section can be quite confusing. I'm not saying this because I failed my listening section (*don't give me that look sistuh!!!*)

Yes, it was the listening section that reduced my band score. But I believe with constant practice anyone can excel at it. Thankfully, I registered for another one and I passed my first stage of the relocation process.

The next stage, acing your IELTS Exam is the CBT Test. I enquired about the CBT and registered for it. CBT requires NMC authorization to book your exam. I got the NMC authorization and registered via one of the approved exam centers in Lagos. The CBT is multiple exam types for four hours. The questions were a bit easy for me, as they have to do with the things one would have a common knowledge of. I also joined few CBT groups that helped with questions and practice. I got my result at midnight the following day. I passed. I aced the second stage of my relocation, and my only song from that day until I left for UK was "Nearer the UK to thee, nearer to thee."

The Role of an Agent in the Relocation Process

Another important stage in the relocation process is getting an agent. This is a very important stage of the relocation process. There are lots of agencies out there and as a result you may get confused on which one is the genuine one. Once you get a genuine agency, the work is half done. It's very important to be careful about the agency you choose for your relocation plan, especially if you are relocating abroad to work as a nurse. I used a different agency, but at a time I had to settle with MMA agency.

MMA is a very popular agency when it comes to helping foreign nurses relocate to their choice of country. It was MMA that helped with my current job. They helped with every other relocation process that had got to do with sourcing for jobs. You have to download a base camp if you are opting with MMA recruitment agency. This is where they give you a detailed process of everything you are going to do in your relocation plans.

Interestingly, MMA has a group on Telegram that helps you prepare for your CBT (MMA CBT GROUP). Once you have selected your choice of Agency, get linked with every one of their activities and start submitting your documents. Before submitting your documents, you have to pay an application fee to get access to the NMC online. The agency helps you apply for jobs. And once you get accepted into any institution you will be called up for an interview. MMA recruitment helped me with applying for jobs and I got a job offer with a healthcare home and was called up for an interview.

The next stage after my interview is to apply for verification by NMC Nigeria. After verification, NMC Nigeria sends your transcript to NMC UK. However, it took a month for NMC Nigeria to conclude my verification. My place of employment in the UK gave me my certificate of sponsorship, which I used in applying for a visa.

The next exam is the OSCE, which should be taken within a few months after coming to the UK. If you are coming to the UK to work as a nurse, the OSCE exam is very essential, as it is what will provide you with your nursing pin.

The nursing pin is a combination of letters and numbers that you get after writing the OSCE exam. The nursing pin is just like the nursing license of Nigeria, which requires you to work anywhere as a nurse in the UK. The OSCE exam is usually sponsored by your employer and everything provided for you as regards preparation.

I got my visa in two weeks and was ready to go live out my dreams in the UK. It's very important to note that this particular process of relocation differs with agencies and comes with the season.

In conclusion, the above was my experience and the processes I used for mine. It's important to make your research about the processes of your agency. Additionally, while you are trying to get information and enquire about a lot of things, some people would take time to respond to you. Family and friends in the country of your choice may seem to hoard information from you, but it's a different thing entirely. I once resented most of them, because I thought they didn't want to give me information. But my experience here has taught me never to judge them. Some of them barely have time and they go through a lot of stress. It is very important to appreciate them when they do give their time to your requests.

Summary of the Step-by-step of Becoming a United Kingdom Registered Nurse (UKRN)

- Get an international passport.

- Preferably write and pass IELTS/OET before starting the process, as it is presumed to be the most challenging of all. IELTS (about 75k); Minimum of Listening- 7.0; Writing- 6.5; Reading- 7.0; Speaking- 7.0. Overall - 7.0. Occupation English Test (OET), which is about 587 AUD currently - Minimum of Reading – B; Writing - C+; Listening – B, and Speaking- B.

- Open an account with NMC UK via *online.nmc-uk.org*

- Pay £140 (you can pay directly yourself with a MasterCard) after filling in the required information. At this stage, you need to upload the data page of your international passport, certificate (notification can be used here if your certificate isn't available yet) and IELTS/OET result (optional at this point). You'll have a personalized NMC portal through which you can monitor your progress all through the whole registration process.

- Pay #17,500 on remittal (pay online if you are outside Abuja and someone is to submit for you. But if in Abuja, you can pay online or in a bank). Alongside evidence of payment, send the photocopies of the following documents to Nursing and Midwifery Council, Nigeria (NMCN) Office; Notification/Certificate, License (front and back), Letter requesting for verification and good standing (you must include your CRM number here;). This CRM number can be found at the top left corner of the mail NMC UK sends after you must have paid

£140. The letter should be addressed to NMCN and should include your name and the exact thing you want i.e., verification and good standing with NMC UK as well as Birth certificate.
- ➤ Wait to be verified and get an authorization test email from Pearson (the organization that handles the CBT exam) to book CBT. Book the CBT (£83) and write the exam. You can buy a voucher for this on https://www.mindhub.co.uk/. You will get a voucher code within 24-48 hours, which you can input when you get to the payment stage of your CBT booking on Pearson site.
- ➤ Fill the final form by NMC UK, which includes an upload of name of medical regulator, police clearance, notification/certificate and IELTS (academics)/OET result (without this, you can't progress beyond this stage. Furthermore, you must have the expected bands, among others).
- ➤ Pay the final registration fee of £153 to NMC UK. This is needed so that you can get your pin from NMC UK (this pin is more like a license to practice). Wait to have good standing done by NMCN (You don't need to pay for this, because the #17,500 covers it).
- ➤ You can start looking for a job at any stage. But preferably, start searching for jobs after you must have passed CBT and IELTS/OET. You can either get an agent or apply directly on **nhs.jobs, tracjobs and indeed.co.uk** for jobs in National Health Service (NHS) hospitals. For care homes, apply on http://www.carehome.co.uk. The benefits for care home vs. NHS vary; choosing one depends on what you want. Try researching on both before making a choice. Generally, care homes are believed to pay more, but NHS hospitals are better for career advancement. Alternatively, you can send emails to some trusts to show interest in working for them.
- ➤ After getting an offer you sign the offer letter and send your

documents to the trust. Note that when you apply directly, you might have to fund your visa and ticket yourself; you get a refund on getting to the UK (this isn't always the case, though). Agents, on the other hand, pay for these upfront. Just ensure you read your offer letter well to know what the trust is offering. The choice is all yours to make at the end of the day.

It's very important to note that the steps above are the most recent steps and may alter depending on when or what year you decide to start your application process.

Another route of working as a nurse in the UK is applying to any university of your choice for masters in adult nursing (pre-registration). It's a two year programme that enables you to be taught and trained to practice as a nurse in the UK. Students who successfully complete this programme will be admitted into the NMC register to practice as registered nurses.

In order to achieve this, you have to be a graduate with at least a 2:1 in your first degree on any course. You will also require sitting for the exam in order to achieve the band score required for IELTS- the English language proficiency exam. This is mainly for international students from countries that do not have English as their main language. This is quite a straight forward process, if you are able to provide all the requirements. Another good part is that you are allowed to work for 20 hours a week as a student. This will help pay your bills at least.

CHAPTER THREE

CHALLENGES OF RELOCATION

Hammers and bricks can break bones, but lack of funds can make relocation hard!

A lot of people are looking forward to relocating abroad for different valid reasons. Young people top the list of aspiring immigrants, and most of them may be unemployed or underpaid. However, relocating abroad for any reason involves spending MONEY. As a Nigerian who has got first-hand experience, you will sure need money to work out your relocation- from registering for your IELTS, CBT, passport, applying for a visa, self-care, and flight preparation. I must reiterate that you will spend money.

Lack of funds was almost a major setback in my plans of relocation. My salary and all my savings at that time weren't enough.

I had to look out for another source of income. Miraculously, a particular patient who had given birth to a set of premature twins that I had nursed before offered me the opportunity to be their home nurse. I grabbed the opportunity with both hands, and luckily for me the pay I got doing this work in a few months' time, as a home nurse, helped in funding my relocation processes.

POSSIBLE CHALLENGES OF MIGRATION PROCEDURES/PREPARATION

1. **Failure to Plan:** You must have a plan before embarking on any relocation procedure. Why do you want to relocate? What steps do you look for while applying for these procedures? Planning gives you an edge and keeps you focused on your goal. However, there can always be a shift in plans, but the fact remains that you made an effort to plan.

2. **Insufficient Funds:** You need funds for any relocation plans. You will spend lots of money, especially if you are planning from Nigeria. What most people who aspire to relocate abroad don't know is the fact that even if you are going for a scholarship abroad, you still need a lot of money to sponsor your travel arrangements. I ran out of money countless times while going about my relocation plans. And it was just the first stage, which involves registering and writing for exams. My job as a nurse, which was my only source of income then, was not enough. I had to start thinking about another source of income, and God did it for me by introducing that new mother I previously mentioned somewhere above. If there is any major problem that anyone could face in the process of relocation plans, it would be lack of finance to prosecute your plans.

3. **Examination/Interviews:** These are important parts of

migration, especially when you are relocating as a professional worker. There are series of exams and interviews that you must undergo. Most of the interviews are unexpected, as you don't even know who you will meet at the interview panel or the questions you would be asked. I was tensed during the first phase of my interview. I experienced some form of palpable excitement and the pressure to impress on the day of interview. To be frank, all of that can be overwhelming for the first time. You may flop if caution is not taken.

The tension and pressure that come with the phase of writing series of exam are a major challenge, because you need to ace your exams to get through other stages.

4. **Travel Preparation:** Travel preparation includes applying for Visa, getting your passport (if you don't have one) and going for series of tests (medical and physical tests). The stress and money involved in these processes are second to none. You need to prepare your mind for this stage, as it can get frustrating at some point. A lot of travelers have faced challenges whenever they apply for a Visa or even attempt to book air tickets. Getting your passport is never enough; you have to still go through the process of Visa application. Things can turn out awful when it comes to getting your visa. You may be rejected or delayed. The most annoying part that you have to deal with is the Nigerian immigration services that may cause the increase in the delay of your Visa.

5. **Delay from Agencies:** After submitting the required documents and information to my agency, I was expecting a swift reply from them, but there was no reply from them for a long time. I kept getting, "We will get back to you," and it was already few months till my supposed departure date. I kept hearing, 'No reply!' 'No calls!' 'No emails!' I can vividly remember refreshing my email

twenty times every day in hope of getting mails from them, but to no avail. Nothing has ever been comparably frustrating!

However, the best part was that I had already bought the things I needed for my departure: clothes and food stuff! Lol! But why shouldn't I? That was the first phase of the procedure, and I was supposed to leave in few months. Because I am a proactive person, I started buying things on time, but ended up eating all of them because of the delay. I know you are laughing right now, *lol...*

Do you know the saying, "Delay is dangerous"? *This was it!!!* And it can be frustratingly dangerous. But the good news is you will always have options. I had options, but one thing with having options is making the best choice. I had the option of going with NHS, but I had weighed their criteria and it wasn't aligning with what I wanted. And to worsen the matter, their pay was lesser. It wasn't easy for me as I almost accepted NHS, until God intervened and I got an email from my agency. Voila!!!

Now, everything seems scary, right?!! You are a bit shaken! Yea, I know that feeling. And at this point you are wondering if you can go through all of these challenges. How do you overcome them? Well, as long as you are still holding this book in your hand, you will get through all of the processes. I will show you how I did mine and succeeded.

CHAPTER FOUR

THE SILVER LINING

"Hope is being able to see that there is light despite all the darkness"
- Desmond Tutu.

Failure is a mindset. One thing about failure is that it can wipe away memories of previous successes and achievements. It is capable of reminding you of your incapability and weaknesses. Unless we see failure as an opportunity to begin again intelligently, it will remain an immovable barrier in our lives. The truth is that failure is never the end of the road, but simply an indicator that there are areas in our lives where we need to put more efforts in order to actualize our desired results or goals.

I failed my IELTS on my first attempt. Naturally, in the wake of the failure I struggled with overcoming the thoughts of failure. Many questions kept popping up in my head: What if I register and fail again? What if I will never pass IELTS? The *"what ifs"* didn't stop and I almost got discouraged. But I had to try again. The truth is that we would never know what would happen unless we try. It only takes an *"umph"* for anyone to tri*umph,* only if they try.

The fear of failure and the sorrows that come from failing have kept a lot of dreams short-lived and unrealized.

When I got my IELTS result for my first attempt and saw that I scored below the expected band, I was truly devastated. But what could I do? I registered again! When the negative *"What if"* questions came popping up in my head days after I got the result, I decided to turn them into positive *"what if"* questions. The positive questions became, "What if I didn't register and miss my chance of achieving my dreams"? What if I pass the exams on my second attempt? What if this is my chance? These questions helped me in finding courage to register for another IELTS exam, which I eventually passed. The section where I failed in my first attempt was the listening section. To be honest, it was partly my fault because I lost concentration at some point and couldn't get through with the passage.

The Power of Perseverance
Finally, I registered for another IELTS, and this time I practised more than before. I worked on my concentration level by listening to more podcasts and also listened attentively to people to get everything they said within a particular time frame. I identified all the loopholes and intensified my practice. I still studied with my previous YouTube tutors, but most importantly, I kept submitting my practical questions to professionals via emails for assessments. I spent more time improving my listening skills and catching up of words. I wrote my second IELTS examination some months after I failed at the first attempt and passed comfortably. I aced every section and scored 8.5! Consequently, the burst of joy and gratitude I experienced on that fateful day was so overwhelming, as I saw the first stage of my dream coming into reality – *checkmate!!!*

After acing my second IELTS, I proceeded to the next stage of CBT and the series of interviews that followed. In the previous chapter,

I wrote about the delays I encountered after I had submitted the required documents. The delay in response from my agency almost cost me my peace and dreams. So many disturbing thoughts kept coming to my minds, and I began questioning God's will for my life. I began wondering and asking: maybe this was not what God wanted for me. I was saying, maybe I am not worthy of better things, etc. Once you start experiencing a delay like this or on any project, there will be influx of doubts coming to your mind to affect negatively your authenticity and your self-worth.

Delay usually comes with a temptation to accept the available choice, and it happened to me. What I did was that, I held onto God and the assurance of my internal validation. I believed: *I'm worth it!* And I would get whatever I worked for. These were my assurances, supported with prayers, and the delay was broken. What do you do when you experience delay? How do you hold on till the end?

The following tips helped me during my delay period. I hope they would help you too:

1. **Hold on to your belief:** Never stop believing in yourself and in God. Delay comes with self-doubt and anxiety. Doubt will make you to constantly question your abilities and despise or undermine your strengths. But this is the time to hold onto who you are. Think about how far you've come and your small wins. What have you achieved before now? Take a moment and enjoy your little victories.

2. **Ask questions:** Delay is not a period where you stop asking questions. When I experienced a delay with my agency, I went to ask for other options and their requirements. I asked my friends who have passed through this phase and how they overcame the phase. Asking questions in the time of delay helps you know whether you are wasting your time waiting.

3. **Don't get stuck:** Honestly, I almost got stuck while waiting for my agency. The delay was taking too long and the supposedly second option had a close deadline. So, I was stuck between continuing waiting or giving up on my agency. The pressure was overwhelming, but because I had already asked questions about my second option it made me weigh the best option and stayed for the best. You may get stuck when you are experiencing delay, to put it mildly. But then, you have to think of the options that are best for you. Is it better to wait or choose the other option and forever get stuck with something you will regret the rest of your life?

4. **Be Patient:** Patience is always the key. Impatience can lead you to make regrettable decisions and it will be difficult to pick up the pieces. Think of trying to fix a broken glass. If you succeed in it, be sure it would never look the same. Be patient in your pursuit to achieve your goals. Nothing beats patience in time of delay.

5. **Avoid hasty decisions:** Never try to act based on your emotions. I understand this is a moment where your emotions are all over the place and you cannot control them. But do not make decisions when you are emotional. Be sure of your next step and do not make a move because you are tired of waiting. Weigh your decisions extensively.

6. **Pray:** Prayer gives you the strength you need to keep with delay of any sort. Prayer hastens the processes and assures you that you will get what you want. Don't stop praying and asking God to give you the strength to be patient enough for his will to be done in your life.

7. **Take care of yourself:** Do not neglect your physical, spiritual, and mental health. A lot of people tend to neglect

their overall wellbeing as they go through a rough phase in their lives, and expectedly, the result of the neglect will be seen at some point in their lives. The aftermath of your negligence can be terrible and may prevent you from enjoying the fruits of your patience.

8. **Beware of Promises:** This is a point where you get lots of promises from different people. You will encounter people who will tell you to stop waiting because they have a better option for you. Be on your guard before you accept their promises. A lot of friends kept promising a lot of things and it was with good intentions. But I knew what I wanted and the fickleness of human promises, so I kept waiting and I got what I wanted eventually.

Always believe in yourself, be patient, and lean on God in times of trouble. The joy that comes in the morning is greater than the sorrows of the night. You cannot imagine the joy I had when I was finally called and was given the job I wanted. It was dream come true for me. As I stepped my feet on the sand of the country of my residence, having left Nigeria, I knew my life was about to take another direction for good.

CHAPTER FIVE

THE NESTING PHASE

"You will never achieve what you are capable of if you are too attached to the things you need to let go" -Anonymous.

Nothing can be as exciting as seeing your dreams coming to pass. All my life, I've always wanted to be at the top of my career and excel in whatever I decided to do with my life. Stepping my feet on this foreign soil that would give me the platform to soar higher was the beginning of my excellence. After passing through every procedure and landed a job with a care home, my employer booked a connecting flight from Dubai to Glasgow. So, I went en route from Lagos to Dubai and then to Glasgow. Altogether, it was an 18-hour flight and the most tiring journey I've experienced all my life. But honestly, I didn't care. Like!!! This was all I ever wanted and thought for and it was coming to pass right before me. My flight from Lagos to Dubai was at about 4 am and we had to wait till 7am to board the connecting flight to Glasgow.

Do you know what they say about meeting your helper in unexpected places? *Yea!* It came through for me. I met Mrs. O. during my flight and she has become more than a friend to me in Glasgow. How I met Mrs. O. was predestined by God: I was sitting quietly and engrossed in a movie as we waited for the flight to take off when the air hostess came to me and pleaded that I moved to the next seat for a woman who was almost having an asthmatic attack as a result of her present sitting position. I immediately obliged and moved on to the next seat. The woman having taking a seat next to me started coughing, and I immediately asked for water on her behalf. We kicked off from there and started talking. It was in the course of our discussion that I got to know she is a British Citizen originally from South Africa. She told me a lot of things about herself and offered guidelines on how best I would cope in the UK. From all indications, God brought Mrs. O. into my life at the right time and she has been more than a blessing to me. I will also not forget the assistance of my friends, Sam and Kelvin who together with Mrs. O. helped me with some of the basic things I had to do before settling down for work. *They advised and assisted me with opening a bank account, registering GP, and adding my name to the electoral register. These are the first and important things you have to do once you arrive in the UK or any country.*

LIFE IN GLASGOW

My first experience in the UK was not the best. One thing we were not told about relocation asides from the excitement was the loneliness and the culture we must encounter. When I was in Nigeria and my friends would talk about it, I didn't take them seriously, but now I can see everything. The loneliness and cultural shock are real and comes to you like a flash of lightning. No warning! No pep talks! I think people should start speaking up on the loneliness that comes with relocation, because most times the loneliness can be unknowingly depressing. My life in the UK began immediately after I had resumed work two days after my arrival. I missed my bus on my first day and I had to befriend Google Maps to get to my workplace. Luckily, it was just a 25-minute walk to my workplace. I was introduced to my team and afterward was posted to an advanced dementia unit to work in healthcare for the time being, till I got my nursing pin.

Challenges of Settling in a New Country

Settling in a new country poses many challenges. There are common experiences of immigrants across the globe.

Below are top common challenges you are likely to face while trying to settle in a new country.

1. **Cultural Shock:** Think about the fact that you are coming from an entirely different region and you have known only your country. There are a lot of things you would encounter in a foreign region that you have never come across before. These experiences usually come with a shock. I had my first cultural shock when I missed the bus to work and had to walk all the way to my workplace for the first day. Luckily for me, it was just a 25-minute walk. The bus system in Scotland has been designated for different set times. So, if a bus is to leave in particular set time, you will have to wait for the next bus going to the same place to arrive at that bus stop.

2. **Language Barriers**: Language tops the list of issues faced by immigrants in any country. It's usually the first thing you will experience even as a Nigerian coming from an English-speaking country. I also experienced some language barriers with the Scottish people. They speak English with an accelerated and twisted accent; it's a kind of speaking Igbo or Yoruba but with a different dialect. I adapted to the Scottish style of speaking by closely reading their lips and asking some people to take it slowly while having conversations.

3. **Ethical Shock:** Another shock I experienced was in my work place-in addressing your senior colleagues in your

workplace by their names. Back in Nigeria, especially in the healthcare sector, senior colleagues are addressed by "Ma" or "Sir," but when I came to the UK I heard my colleagues addressing the superior manager by her name. Honestly, I had to practice such ethics in front of a mirror on how to call my Boss 'Celine.'

4. **Housing:** Securing a house is a big priority for anybody moving to a new area or country, particularly if a person has no plans beforehand. Although an apartment was already prepared for me before I arrived in the UK, the problem I had with housing was when it was time to find a place for my family. If you are looking forward to inviting your family to join you, know that there is a law that you must get a reasonable and comfortable apartment based on the number of people you wish to accommodate.

5. **Cultural Differences:** Cultural differences range from social customs to more significant issues such as attitudes towards gender, ethnicity, sexuality, and religious adversities, which are all different from what I already knew. Accepting different values does not mean you have to take them as your own, but means that you must respect them.

6. **Discrimination:** Discrimination will certainly be dominant in most places. Discrimination on the grounds of racism is mostly what you have to face as a person of color. Do not let this get to you or reduce your self-esteem. Be unbeatable!

7. **Isolation/Loneliness:** Loneliness is real especially when you are coming from a structure with a strong communal living and support system. Living without the support of close friends and family is a big factor. You will feel so lost and alienated from a lot of things if that

is your case. All things being equal, if a country where individualism is mostly practiced over communal living–operation mind your business in place- you will find yourself disoriented most of the time. I almost suffered chronic depression during my first few months in the UK coupled with Covid-19 restrictions. It was not really a very good experience.

8. **Weather:** I can't tell you how cold it is here until you experience it. When I hear stories of the cold in foreign countries, I assumed it to be like our Harmattan season. Nah! Harmattan doesn't come close to winter. This is not a challenge to overlook, especially if you are coming from a country like mine. The weather may disrupt a lot of your activities for the day, if not properly taken care of.

WORK CHALLENGES

If you have ever worked as a nurse in Nigeria, you would understand that you are not always attached to a particular patient, because you may just meet them once in your care. It's always like-go to work, do your job well, and go home. This is not the same with Nursing homes. There is a rarefied attachment that comes with working in a home: you get attached to your patient and become almost everything to them. In nursing homes, patients depend on their nurses and their 'careers' for everything, and as a result, a special kind of bond is formed or developed between the patient and the staff. I was posted to the advanced dementia unit and I worked there for few months.

Dementia is a condition that damages the brain cells at a certain age. It affects the sufferer's memory, language, problem-solving, and thinking abilities. Those mostly at risk of Dementia are the aged and alcoholics. The condition brings a decline in their normal life activities. Sufferers of dementia may resort to self-harm or become victims of abuse by others, if they are not properly taken care of. My experience in the dementia unit taught me a lot of things.

The most important lesson I learned was gratitude. There are lots of things that we are not grateful for: getting to lift a cup to our mouth, just holding a simple conversation, etc. We get to see our loved ones and hold memorable conversations with them. We laugh, eat and enjoy life with people we care about. Time may come when we may no longer be able do all these things. Every day is the best day to show gratitude for all you are and will ever have. The dementia unit experience was memorable for me. I got my pin after working as a care assistant for few months in the Dementia ward, and to be honest, the experiences gathered in the unit were worth it.

PROFESSIONAL EXAMS AND COVID-19

No one ever envisaged coming into a new country and tucked in lockdown for some good reasons. Coming to a new country should be a moment for adventures and discoveries, a time to move around and feel everything about your new place. I dreamt of going to a lot of places and having fun in my life. We all prepared for 2020, energized by our New Year resolutions, but then Covid-19 came upon the earth suddenly and the world stood still because of the sweeping devastation it came with. Prior to COVID-19, many people hardly knew anything about it. It came against the background of me fulfilling my dream of relocation and starting a new life.

The blow of Covid-19 went hard on me as it was also this period that I was supposed to write my OSCE that would give me my nursing pin and finally qualify me to work as a Nurse in the UK. Universities and businesses were all shut down and I couldn't book for my exam. My original plan was to write my OSCE and then make way for my family to join me. It was not supposed to take too long. Lectures and studies had to be done online. The exams were postponed till further notice. Everything was on hold as people were only struggling to stay alive in the least.

This was the moment my depression set in. I stayed for almost a year without going out and without my family. I was constantly thinking of what would happen next, and asking myself maybe the world was coming to an end. I almost regretted leaving my family. My husband was a strong support system during these periods. We talked every day via WhatsApp video and chats; we prayed and had conversations on lots of issues which, no doubt, helped me manage the depression and isolation satisfactorily. I also kept in touch with my parents, siblings, and friends, and they all helped me through the lockdown and that helped me to a great extent to fight off mental breakdown.

Due to the increased cases of Covid-19, the pressure at work became overbearing and shifts were doubled. Most staff was affected by Covid–19 and that resulted in a decrease in healthcare workers, which further increased work pressure and stress. By the time I was done with a 12-hour shift, I was already exhausted and wouldn't have to finish other things. At some point, my line manager resigned, leaving an avalanche of workload for me. Most of my other colleagues were not as supportive and I was overburdened with work. I also got promoted temporarily to work as a Covid-19 register for oversea nurses in their final registration stages. The promotion allowed me to work as a registered nurse but with restrictions.

Coupled with the lockdown and the workload, my family couldn't come down to me as planned. This was a major factor that caused me depression, as I had to save up money with support from my husband for them to come over. I thought I would never see my family again. I thought the world was coming to an end, or maybe inter-travel would be banned forever. I was helpless!!! But God came through for me, and that was the beginning of my healing journey. Also, meeting Pastor R through a colleague was a huge blessing at that time of my life. God knew I needed someone to lean on, and He divinely arranged Pastor R Through a charity organisation she works with, I got vouchers for food during these difficult times. The way people bought and stored food items as soon as they got the news of going into lockdown was shocking and the same time funny. On a certain evening, after close from work, I went to a superstore close by to get something to eat for dinner, but there was almost no food left on the shelves! chaii!. I was saved by Kelvin who had to take me in his car to another superstore some miles away from my location. Interestingly, God did not just send Pastor R; He also introduced Mrs. P who was my colleague. She made sure I had food throughout the lockdown. She was always there with her bubbling aura and her kind words. I met lots of wonderful and kind people throughout my stay in the UK. I will not go on without mentioning Mummy J who kept encouraging me and my auntie Katie who was also my previous boss. You don't need to go to theatre to listen to any comedian, Katie is gifted to make people laugh and she has a golden heart. l love you all to the moon. Everyone I met was always ready to offer help to me. When I came in at first, I never expected to get more from people in a foreign land, but I was constantly surrounded by the best people who made life easier and less depressing for me.

Sometimes we hold ourselves back from seeking help or embracing kindness. Sometimes too we are lost in thought that we begin to think we are never enough. As you give kindness, dare to take back kindness. Accept kindness from other people, agree to lean and cry on shoulders that offer solace, bask in the love and care of people around you. Don't hold anything in, let it out. Accepting genuine kindness and love does not make you lose your strength. *Breathe!!!*

CHAPTER SIX

TURNING POINT

"Trust in the Lord with all your heart. Do not try to figure out anything on your own..." – Proverbs 3:5

You know that popular saying; "When life gives you lemons, make lemonades." Now, the question is, What if you don't want lemonade? What if you are allergic to lemonade? One thing about the universe is that it listens to our vibration energies. The Universe understands our desires and agrees to the desires that will make our life better and happy. Most times people confuse this as the will of God, but God also listens to us and is an ardent promoter of self-belief and self-validation. God shows you options to make sure you know what you want. God wants to grant our expectations. That's His thought for us! So, when life gives you lemons, demand for apples, if that's what you want. You will surely get it.

As the lockdown was slowly coming to an end as some part of the world began to open its doors, people were allowed to come out but with strict adherence to set precautions. I was finally able to register for my OSCE and attended training via zoom. The exam was written in England. When the result came out, I failed a station. I was almost dead because of the result. I felt terrible. I lost hope. It felt like my dreams were beginning to fall apart. I felt *"my village people"* were after me. I shared this with almost anyone that cares to listen. It was my moment of absolute surrender, when all chips were down. It was indeed the moment when I felt helpless. I am a strong and resilient woman to the best of my knowledge, but I must admit that at this moment I reached a breaking point.

The challenges I faced seemed to want to swallow me. One night, after close of work, I was walking home and thinking at the same time, pointing out one after another, what was facing me and the shame ahead of me. You can imagine me thinking of the shame instead of the victory ahead. This is what happens when you feel overpowered and have lost trust in God. When I failed my OSCE, lock down palaver, work challenges, loneliness, family responsibilities and lack of clarity in all... hmm! I kept listing as I walked on the lonely path and at this point, I broke down in uncontrollable tears.

That night I got home and laid on my bed and played the song titled, *"Way maker by the Gospel Artist Sinach,"* and then God whispered to me through the song. He spoke to me. I felt Him. It was very real! He asked me to open my Bible to Proverbs 3:5...and I read from the message translation. That night I will never forget. It was a moment of absolute surrender and rekindling of my trust in God, who is concerned about me and can do all things. God came through for me again in Glasgow! My path was lightened up again and I continued in my journey with much strength.

Immediately after that encounter, I applied for a re-sit and I doubled my preparations. With the help of God, a much more focused preparation, and the encouragement of wonderful women of God I passed my re-sit and within two days I was moved to the permanent register, received my pin, and I became a registered nurse in the UK. No moment has ever been surreal! All my hard works have finally paid off. I felt so proud on the day my name was being moved to the register. This was what I wanted. I demanded for apples-big red ones- worked hard for it, backed by patience, prayers, consistency, and I got what I wanted in the end. I am continuing to register success in my life and career.

Just one year after, I was promoted to manage one of the nursing units in my place of employment. I am not ashamed to say it was by the hand of God! Metamorphosed from a young girl who was once unsure about what was really ahead of her but was relentless in pursuing her dreams into a young woman on the ladder of success. I would say I am not yet where I want to be, but surely with God on my side I am getting there. I am looking forward to a greater me as I journey with God in life.

MY ENCOURAGEMENT
Dear reader,
What are you going through right now as you are reading this book?
What is your aspiration or expectations?
Do you seem lost in this journey of life?
What demand have you placed on life?
What is life actually giving to you?
Do you feel that you are not enough?
I want to encourage you not to give up your faith. Life is a journey full of potholes, but with determination and trust in God you will surely arrive at your destination. Always pray to meet the right people in your journey. Do not just accept anything that life dishes to you; you have authority to place a demand on life. Get trainings, develop yourself and always be the best of yourself, wherever you find yourself.

CHAPTER SEVEN

FAMILY REUNION

I was prepared for my family to come over, months after the lockdown was eased and I had gotten a new place. I got a new apartment and everything was set to welcome them. Inviting your family over is not difficult as long there are funds available to sponsor all documentations and tickets. My husband was supportive and within few months everything was ready. Reuniting with my family has been one of the happiest moments of my life in the UK. That joy of holding your kids after so many months and moments of helplessness could not be bought. And as John Wooden would say, "The most important thing in the world is Family and love."

TIPS FOR ASPIRING YOUNG NURSES LOOKING FORWARD TO WORKING ABROAD (and anyone desiring success)

1. **Decide:** Making the decision that you want to work abroad is the first step. You have to sit down and decide what you want. Ask yourself certain questions and be

ready to follow up your decisions with actions that can move you forward to your goal.

2. **Plan:** Nothing beats planning ahead of time. Planning helps you stay focused. Once you have decided to work abroad, start planning on every possible and legal thing to do to make it work. Ask questions, use the internet, check videos on YouTube and make acquaintances with people already working abroad.

3. **Save:** I want to scream this in particular from the rooftop. I can't explain how important saving for a project like this is. You need money! I will advise you start now and save money.

4. **Pray:** At every step of your application, pray. Tell God about it and ask for divine intervention, conviction and discernment.

5. **Connect:** Connect with people of like minds. Find people who are also interested in working abroad and form a discussion/plan group. Working with like minds will give you the encouragement and all the positive vibes you need.

6. **Start studying early enough:** This is very important, especially when you are looking forward to writing your IELTS and other professional exams you will come across. Don't wait till one week before the exam before you begin to hustle for materials. ***Start now!***

CONCLUSION

Nothing good comes easy, but with hard work and good preparation we can achieve our dreams. Naysayers and challenges may arise, but we must keep standing tall. I have arrived at a certain point in my pursuit of success and I am poised to achieve more. Every experience and tip I have shared in this book has helped to shape my life as regards achieving my plans.

The journey wasn't always rosy, but I made it and I believe anyone can make it to this point. You just have to get up and act. Don't be comfortable with mediocrity. Do not accept the standards that have been set to keep you stagnant. If you are not comfortable or happy with your present situation, do something to change it for good. Run if you can't fly. Walk if you can't run. Crawl if you can't walk. You just have to get up and make a move in your life, for nothing good comes easy. There will always be a way.

May you find the encouragement and the resources needed for a better, healthier and happier life. Everything good will come to you in the end.

For Enquiries contact:
Email nzlizzy@gmail.com

ABOUT THE AUTHOR

Chinazo Elizabeth Egwuh

Chinazo is a Nigeria- Trained registered nurse currently practicing in the United Kingdom.

She is a Christain and married with two wonderful kids.